HERBAL REMEDIES FOR RESTLESS LEGS SYNDROME

Discover Holistic Healing: Effective Solutions To   Soothe And Alleviate Lasting Relief

DR. JEREMY ALLEY

Copyright © DR. JEREMY ALLEY 2024

All rights reserved. No part of this publication may be reproduced, distributed, or transmitted in any form or by any means, including photocopying, recording, or other electronic or mechanical methods, without the prior written permission of the author, except in the case of brief quotations embodied in critical reviews and certain other noncommercial uses permitted by copyright law.

Disclaimer:

The information provided in this book, is intended for general informational purposes only and should not be considered as professional advice.

The author has made every effort to ensure the accuracy of the information presented. However, readers are advised to consult with a qualified healthcare professional before attempting any herbal remedies or making significant changes to their wellness routine. Individual health conditions vary, and what may be suitable for one person may not be appropriate for another.

It is important to note that the author is not in any endorsement deal, partnership, or affiliation with any organization, brand, or company mentioned in this book. Any references to specific products or services are based on the author's personal experience or general knowledge and do not imply an endorsement or promotion of those products or services.

Contents

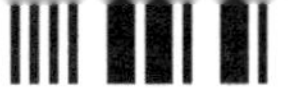

Overview

It might be difficult to control restless legs syndrome (RLS), which frequently causes discomfort and interferes with day-to-day activities. The purpose of this tutorial is to investigate herbal medicines as a substitute method of treating the symptoms of restless legs syndrome. By being aware of the subtleties of RLS and the possible advantages of using herbal remedies, people can improve their general health and experience alleviation.

About The Book

This is a thorough investigation of herbal treatments for restless legs syndrome. This guide focuses on natural remedies that may help with symptom relief to offer insightful information about alternate methods of controlling RLS. We must approach herbal treatments with an open mind as we embark on this path, acknowledging the various ways that nature's gifts might improve our health.

RLS: A Synopsis of Restless Legs Syndrome

Understanding Restless Legs Syndrome fundamentally is essential before exploring natural therapies. RLS is a neurological condition marked by an overwhelming need to move the legs, frequently accompanied by tingling, itching, or painful pains. These symptoms usually get worse when people are idle, especially at night or in the evening, which makes it difficult for them to unwind and get a good night's sleep.

Although the precise etiology of RLS is still unknown, factors like pregnancy, iron deficiency, heredity, and several drugs have been connected to the start of the condition. Understanding how complicated this illness is sets the stage for investigating other methods, such as using herbal remedies, to lessen its effects on day-to-day functioning.

The Value of Herbal Treatments

Herbal treatments are a valuable tool for treating the symptoms of restless legs syndrome since they provide a safe, all-natural method of managing symptoms. Herbal remedies frequently utilize the therapeutic qualities of plants without having negative side effects, in contrast to pharmaceutical interventions that could have unfavorable effects.

Herbal therapies are significant because they can treat the underlying causes of RLS, hence enhancing general health as opposed to just treating symptoms. Numerous herbs have qualities that help improve circulation, lessen inflammation, and encourage relaxation—all of which are important for controlling the discomfort brought on by restless legs syndrome.

Furthermore, taking into account each person's particular needs and sensitivities, herbal therapies frequently offer a more individualized and gentler approach to symptom relief. It is crucial to approach this investigation of different herbs and their possible advantages with knowledge of the complementary nature of herbal medicines in the larger context of health and wellness.

Comprehending the syndrome of restless legs

A neurological condition known as restless legs syndrome (RLS) is typified by an overwhelming need to move the legs and is frequently accompanied by uncomfortable feelings. Although it can affect other regions of the body, this illness mainly affects the legs. RLS patients usually have symptoms when they are sitting or lying down, which can interfere with everyday activities and sleep.

RLS Definition and Symptoms

The primary symptom of restless legs syndrome is an intense need to move the legs, which is typically accompanied by discomfort. People frequently describe these feelings as crawling, tingling, burning, or itching. The symptoms typically get worse in the evening or at night, which affects the affected person's quality of life greatly and causes sleep difficulties.

RLS symptoms can range widely in intensity, from moderate to severe. Some people may only have sporadic discomfort, while others may have chronic agitation.

Reasons and Danger Elements

Although the precise origin of restless legs syndrome is unknown, environmental and genetic factors are thought to be involved. Studies indicate a significant hereditary component, with an

increased risk of getting RLS in families with a history of the disorder. RLS may be exacerbated by several illnesses, including peripheral neuropathy, kidney failure, and iron shortage.

In addition, certain drugs, pregnancy, and hormonal changes might cause or worsen symptoms.

Medical diagnosis and treatment

Finding the cause of restless legs syndrome requires a complete medical history as well as a physical examination. The frequency, type, and possible causes of symptoms may all be questioned by medical professionals. Blood tests may occasionally be performed to look for iron deficiency or other underlying medical issues. RLS has no known cure, although several medicinal interventions can help control symptoms and enhance quality of life. Benzodiazepines, anti-seizure medications, and dopamine agonists are among the medications that are frequently recommended to treat symptoms and encourage improved sleep.

It's crucial to remember that these drugs may not work for everyone and that adverse effects are possible. As supportive measures, lifestyle changes like consistent sleep patterns, regular exercise, and abstaining from coffee and nicotine are frequently advised. Consulting a healthcare provider is essential to establish the best course of action for treating Restless Legs Syndrome in more severe situations where symptoms substantially interfere with everyday functioning.

CHAPTER ONE

USE OF HERBS TO TREAT RESTLESS LEGS SYNDROME

A neurological condition known as restless legs syndrome (RLS) is typified by an overwhelming need to move the legs and is frequently accompanied by uncomfortable feelings. While there are traditional therapies available, some people choose to alleviate their symptoms and encourage better sleep by using herbal medicines. Gaining insight into the benefits of herbal medicines might help determine their possible effectiveness.

Benefits Of Using Herbal Treatments

The natural makeup of herbal therapies for restless legs syndrome is one of its main benefits. Compounds found in many herbs can favorably affect the neurological system, which can aid in reducing the pain and symptoms related to RLS. Furthermore, compared to pharmaceutical options, herbal therapies frequently have fewer side effects, which could make them a safer option for people looking for alternative treatments.

Common Herbs For RLS Therapy

Several herbs have become well-known for their ability to treat restless legs syndrome. These plants can be taken as teas, supplements, or essential oils, among other forms. Investigating these organic choices can reveal more about their possible advantages.

Root Of Valerian

One well-known herb with sedative qualities is Valerian root. It has long been used to encourage calm and enhance the quality of sleep. Valerian root has the potential to alleviate restlessness and pain in those with RLS, thereby offering respite to those who are afflicted. Including valerian root in a nightly regimen could help promote better quality sleep.

a passionflower

Another herb with a reputation for being relaxing is passionflower. It has ingredients that affect the central nervous system in a way that eases tension in the muscles and encourages relaxation. Passionflower may help those suffering from restless legs syndrome by relieving their incessant need to move their legs, which could enhance their sleep patterns.

Lavender

Beyond only being fragrant, lavender offers relaxing qualities. It is commonly known for its pleasant perfume.

Using dried lavender in sachets or pillows, or using lavender essential oil, can help promote relaxation and possibly lessen RLS symptoms.

Chamomile

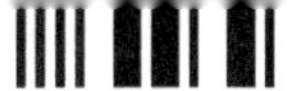

Because of its well-known calming effects, chamomile is frequently used to encourage rest and sleep. Those who suffer from Restless Legs Syndrome may find it easier to relax and lessen their restlessness if they sip chamomile tea before bed.

Others

Several additional herbs have also shown potential in the management of RLS symptoms. These might consist of ginkgo biloba, skullcap, and kava, among others.

People who are thinking about using herbal medicines should speak with medical specialists to be sure they are the right choices for their overall health as well as any ailments they may already have.

For those looking for a natural and maybe successful option to alleviate the pain and restlessness linked to restless legs syndrome, the herbal method presents an opportunity. Individuals might be empowered to make well-informed decisions about integrating herbal treatments into their overall management approach by learning about the benefits and investigating common herbs used in RLS treatment.

CHAPTER TWO

SUSTAINABLE ENVIRONMENT CREATING

Creating a calming atmosphere is essential for people with restless legs syndrome. This entails furnishing the bedroom with a soothing ambiance that encourages rest. Steer clear of over stimuli, such as bright lights and loud noises, to create a more tranquil sleeping environment. Additionally, reducing screen time before bed and sticking to a regular sleep pattern will help RLS patients have better sleep overall.

The Value Of Good Sleep Practices

Keeping up a healthy sleep routine is essential for controlling restless legs syndrome. This entails maintaining a regular sleep schedule, making sure the bedroom is cozy and sleep-friendly, and engaging in relaxing activities before going to bed.

Herbal treatments can promote the promotion of peaceful sleep in addition to these techniques.

Techniques For Relaxation

People with Restless Legs Syndrome may benefit from incorporating relaxing techniques. Herbal therapies that help induce relaxation before bedtime include chamomile tea, which is well-known for its relaxing effects. Comparably, herbs like passionflower and valerian root have long been used to treat restlessness and sleeplessness, which makes them possible friends in the treatment of RLS symptoms.

Establishing A Cozy Sleep Environment

Making a cozy sleeping space requires being aware of things that could make symptoms of restless legs syndrome worse. This entails having cozy bedding, keeping the room cool, and making sure the legs are properly supported. Herbal remedies, such as the calming aroma of lavender essential oil, can be diffused in the bedroom to create a calm environment that promotes relaxation.

Although herbal medicines can help with the management of restless legs syndrome, people should always speak with a healthcare provider before starting any new treatment regimen.

Furthermore, keeping a holistic approach that incorporates lifestyle modifications, natural therapies, and, if required, medical interventions might lead to more successful

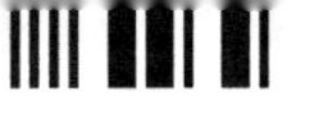

CHAPTER THREE

HERBAL CURES AND CHANGES TO LIFESTYLE

A neurological condition known as restless legs syndrome (RLS) is typified by an overwhelming need to move the legs and is frequently accompanied by uncomfortable feelings. While there are established therapies for RLS, some people choose to address their symptoms using herbal medicines and lifestyle modifications.

Nutritional Modifications For RLS

When it comes to treating restless legs syndrome, nutrition is vital. A few dietary changes could help reduce discomfort. For some RLS sufferers, increasing iron intake—either through supplements or foods high in iron, such as red meat and spinach—has proven advantages. Including foods high in magnesium, such as almonds, bananas, and dark chocolate, may also help with symptom relief.

Because caffeine and nicotine can aggravate RLS symptoms, it might be helpful to cut back on or stop using them. A possible correlation between dietary additives such as artificial sweeteners and monosodium glutamate (MSG) and RLS exacerbation has been suggested by the fact that some people find relief by avoiding them.

Yoga And Exercise To Relieve Stress

Physical activity regularly can help manage the symptoms of RLS. Improved circulation and neurotransmitter regulation are two benefits of exercise for restless legs. Including exercises like swimming, cycling, or walking on a daily schedule may help with symptom relief.

Yoga has also been investigated as an additional strategy for treating RLS because of its emphasis on relaxation and flexibility. For those who struggle with restless legs, there are some yoga poses that work the legs and help with general relaxation.

Some practitioners say that frequent yoga practice helps with better symptoms, while a study in this area is still underway.

Techniques For Stress Management

Anxiety and stress can make symptoms of restless legs syndrome worse. Using stress-reduction strategies could help reduce RLS's physical and psychological symptoms. Techniques like progressive muscle relaxation, deep breathing, and meditation can help induce a more relaxed mental state, which may lessen the severity of restless legs.

For those who have sleep difficulties associated with RLS, developing a nightly regimen that incorporates relaxation techniques might be especially beneficial. Developing a relaxing bedtime routine, such as reading a book or having a warm bath, might improve the quality of sleep and lessen the negative effects of RLS on nocturnal sleep.

Although there may not be a cure for restless legs syndrome, people looking for non-traditional ways to manage their symptoms may find some respite from the condition with the help of herbal medicines and lifestyle modifications. Individuals contemplating these techniques must confer with healthcare experts to guarantee a thorough and customized strategy for managing RLS.

Hygiene Of Sleep

Developing sound sleeping habits is the cornerstone of treating restless legs syndrome. Adopting routines and behaviors that support restful sleep is known as sleep hygiene. The concepts of sleep hygiene are examined in this part, along with practical methods that people with RLS can use to enhance their sleeping environment. For those with RLS, these techniques can help improve their quality of sleep. They range from adhering to a regular sleep schedule to maximizing bedroom settings.

Establishing A Sleep-Friendly Space

Creating a sleep environment that promotes restful sleep is an essential part of controlling restless legs syndrome. This chapter explores the particular steps people might take to create a more cozy and tranquil sleeping environment. Reducing noise, modifying lighting, and selecting the ideal mattress and pillows are just a few ways to make an environment more conducive to sleep for people with RLS.

Creating A Schedule

The secret to controlling RLS symptoms is consistency. The significance of creating a daily routine that encourages relaxation and aids in controlling sleep patterns is emphasized in this section.

Regular exercise, stress management, and relaxing nighttime routines are discussed as essential elements of a regimen designed for those with restless legs syndrome.

Meditation And Mindfulness

People with restless legs syndrome may benefit from practicing mindfulness and meditation. This chapter examines the management of stress and anxiety, which are recognized to be triggers for symptoms of RLS, through techniques including deep breathing exercises and mindfulness meditation.

A general decrease in the symptoms of restless legs syndrome and an improvement in the quality of sleep may result from incorporating these mindful practices into daily living.

This book offers a thorough overview of herbal treatments for RLS, along with insightful advice on how to create a sleep-friendly atmosphere, practice mindfulness and meditation, and maintain good sleep hygiene. People with RLS can try to better control their symptoms and have a more comfortable night's sleep by investigating these natural remedies.

CHAPTER FOUR

TEAS AND RECIPES USING HERBS

An insatiable desire to move the legs is the hallmark of restless legs syndrome (RLS), which is frequently accompanied by uncomfortable feelings.

Those who are looking for natural alternatives may find relief with herbal medicines. Using herbal recipes and teas that capitalize on the medicinal qualities of different plants is one strategy.

Recipes For Herbal Tea

Herbal teas have been used for their calming effects for a very long time, and people with restless legs may find them especially helpful.

For example, chamomile tea has been shown to have relaxing properties and may be able to ease the discomfort that comes with RLS. Before going to bed, making a cup of chamomile tea may help promote relaxation and reduce symptoms.

Another herbal remedy that might help with improving sleep and lowering restlessness related to RLS is Valerian root tea. Due to its sedative qualities, Valerian root is a well-liked option for anyone looking for a natural sleep aid. Including this herbal tea in your nightly ritual could help you get a better night's sleep.

Herbal Infusions To Alleviate RLS

Herbal infusions can be made to address restless legs syndrome in addition to herbal drinks. Infusing passionflower to make a tranquil beverage is a great idea because of its well-known calming and muscle-relaxing effects. Regularly consuming passionflower infusion may help reduce the symptoms of restless legs syndrome (RLS), offering a non-pharmacological alternative for individuals who choose not to use medications.

Lavender can also be added to infusions, giving them a soothing scent. Drinking an herbal tea infused with lavender has long been used to induce relaxation and peace, which may lessen restlessness related to restless leg syndrome (RLS).

Including Herbs In Everyday Meals

Herbal teas and infusions are not the only remedies for restless legs syndrome; adding certain herbs to regular meals can also be a tasty and useful approach.

Due to its anti-inflammatory qualities, turmeric can be included in a variety of recipes. Turmeric may aid people with RLS by reducing inflammation in the body, according to certain research.

Garlic can be added to meals and is well-known for its many health benefits. Although further research is required, there is evidence to suggest that the antioxidant and anti-inflammatory components of garlic may help reduce the symptoms of RLS.

Investigating herbal treatments for restless legs syndrome can be a comprehensive and all-natural way to treat symptoms.

By utilizing the medicinal qualities of these plant-based medicines, people can find solace and peace through the use of herbal teas, infusions, or in their regular meals. Before adding additional herbs or supplements to your regimen, always get medical advice, especially if you have underlying medical conditions or are using other prescriptions.

CHAPTER FIVE

CASE RESEARCH

A neurological condition known as restless legs syndrome (RLS) is typified by an overwhelming need to move the legs and is frequently accompanied by uncomfortable feelings. Examining several case studies is necessary to comprehend how herbal therapies affect RLS. These studies offer insightful information about how herbal therapies have helped people with their RLS symptoms. Scholars and medical professionals have chronicled particular examples to provide insight into how well herbal medicines work to manage and ease the discomfort associated with restless legs syndrome.

Actual Success Stories

A more individualized viewpoint on the usage of herbal treatments for restless legs syndrome can be obtained by looking at real-life success stories. These accounts explore the experiences of people who have effectively included herbal remedies in their regimens for managing RLS.

Success stories demonstrate the effectiveness of herbal therapies and offer insight into the difficulties faced by those with RLS as well as the benefits derived from herbal interventions. These narratives offer motivation and direction to those looking for all-natural ways to manage their RLS symptoms.

First-Hand Accounts Of Herbal Medicine Use

The field of herbal remedies for restless legs syndrome goes beyond research findings and case studies; it also includes firsthand accounts from people who have used herbal remedies to help them through their RLS journey.

These first-person narratives explore the day-to-day difficulties associated with managing RLS and the ways that herbal remedies have positively impacted the lives of those afflicted.

Experiences firsthand provide a nuanced understanding of the usefulness of combining herbal remedies and highlight the comprehensive effects these treatments can have on the general well-being of people suffering from restless legs syndrome.

CHAPTER SIX

SAFETY MEASUREMENTS AND CONTACTS

It's important to think about possible interactions and safety measures before using herbal therapies to treat restless legs syndrome.

The significance of speaking with medical professionals before beginning any herbal regimen is discussed in this section. It highlights how important it is to take a team approach to make sure people make educated decisions regarding their health.

Talking With Medical Professionals

Herbal therapies should not be used in place of expert medical guidance, although they may supplement conventional therapy. The need to speak with medical professionals—such as physicians, neurologists, or specialists

knowledgeable in restless legs syndrome—is emphasized in this section. It promotes candid conversation to develop a comprehensive and unique strategy for managing the illness.

Possible Drug-Herb Interactions

It is crucial to comprehend the possible interplay between herbal medicines and conventional pharmaceuticals to guarantee both safety and effectiveness.

The intricacies of herb-drug interactions are examined in this section, providing insight into how specific herbs may affect the efficacy or security of prescription drugs. People who are knowledgeable in this field are more equipped to make decisions regarding their health.

Guidelines For Dosage And Usage

Herbal medicines, like any form of treatment, require careful consideration of dosage and proper usage. This section includes advice on how to establish the optimum dosage for particular herbs used in controlling Restless Legs Syndrome. It also covers topics like tolerance thresholds, individual variations, and the significance of consistency in getting the best outcomes.

The goal of this book is to provide a thorough overview of herbal treatments for restless legs syndrome. Through the discussion of safety measures, the emphasis on consulting a healthcare provider, the examination of possible interactions, and the provision of dose guidelines, readers can approach herbal remedies with assurance and make well-informed decisions.

CHAPTER SEVEN

RLS AND EXERCISE

Getting moving is essential for controlling RLS symptoms. Frequent exercise has been shown to improve general health and alleviate symptoms.

This section examines the connection between physical activity and restless legs syndrome, emphasizing the kinds of physical activity that may be especially helpful.

Positive Exercises

It's crucial to concentrate on exercises that increase flexibility, relaxation, and circulation when trying to treat RLS with exercise.

This section of the manual explores particular exercises that have demonstrated potential in reducing symptoms associated with restless legs syndrome.

Yoga And Stretches

Yoga and stretches are well-known for encouraging ease and flexibility. This section looks at how a daily regimen that includes yoga and stretching exercises may help manage the symptoms of RLS.

Minimal-Impact Exercises

Low-impact activities offer a more gentle form of exercise for people with RLS. This section of the guide addresses exercises including walking, cycling, and swimming, highlighting how they may help promote leg mobility without aggravating symptoms of RLS.

Healing Techniques

RLS symptoms may improve when restorative techniques like mindfulness and meditation are incorporated. This section examines how mind-body practices might promote relaxation and potentially lessen the discomfort brought on by restless legs syndrome.

Breathing Techniques

Our general sense of peace and well-being might be influenced by the way we breathe. To encourage relaxation and maybe reduce symptoms, people with RLS might adopt the particular breathing techniques covered in this section into their regular practice.

Through the investigation of various herbal remedies and lifestyle changes, people suffering from restless legs syndrome can start a natural, holistic path to managing their problems.

The Prospects Of Botanical Remedies

The integration of herbal treatments into conventional healthcare appears to have exciting prospects in the future, given the growing interest in them. We can make significant progress in our understanding of how these therapies can help with the management of restless legs syndrome by investigating novel herbs and plant-based substances. This section examines how herbal remedies are developing and how they can influence RLS care in the future.

Continued Research

Researchers are continuously examining the safety and effectiveness of different herbs as potential treatments for restless legs syndrome. This section examines the state of the research at the moment, emphasizing studies that investigate the possible advantages of particular herbs in reducing RLS symptoms. People can make educated judgments regarding adding herbal medicines to their RLS treatment plan by keeping up with the latest research.

New Developments In Herbal Medicine

New treatments are constantly developing in the rapidly growing field of herbal medicine, providing novel approaches to the treatment of restless legs syndrome. The most recent herbal treatments that appear to be effective in treating RLS symptoms are covered in this section. Through investigating these new choices, people can remain up to date on the state of herbal remedies and think about integrating them into their customized approach to managing RLS.

For people who want to use herbal therapies as a part of their management plan for restless legs syndrome, this book is a helpful resource. People can make educated judgments about their overall health by receiving knowledge on the state of research, new treatments, and the possible future of herbal remedies.

CONCLUSION

A summary of the most important discoveries and lessons will be given at the end of the guide for readers. The advantages of herbal therapies for restless legs syndrome will be emphasized, and readers will be urged to investigate these natural options as part of a comprehensive strategy for controlling RLS. The purpose of this part is to give readers hope and a sense of empowerment over their ability to use herbal therapies to treat restless legs syndrome.

Summary Of Important Ideas

This section provides a brief synopsis of the main ideas covered throughout the handbook to help reinforce those concepts. This summary, which summarizes key information regarding RLS, its symptoms, and the mentioned herbal treatments, can be used by readers as a quick reference. As they set out on their path to naturally treat restless legs syndrome, readers can refer back to important details with the aid of this summary.

Motivation For Perusers

The book's last portion seeks to uplift readers who are thinking about or have already started, using herbal therapies for RLS. It will provide encouraging words and reaffirm that natural techniques can be beneficial parts of an all-encompassing RLS management strategy. The goal of this encouragement is to give readers confidence so they can make decisions that are best for their health and well-being.